Fun Zen

coloring book

33 coloring pages

by Kate Stevens

Introduction

Nothing gives more pleasure and relaxation than coloring.

It's all about having some time to yourself and creating something unique. You decide the colors, you decide which page to do today and there is no right or wrong way to do it.

You can even cut the page out and frame it as it is!

Most importantly, have fun!

The images can be colored by the whole family.

I truly hope you have enjoyed this book!